LEADING
THE
WAY

LEADING THE WAY

Third Edition

The Busy Nurse's Guide to Supervision in Long-Term Care

Karl Pillemer, Ph.D and

Christine Rheaume, RN

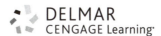

DELMAR
CENGAGE Learning·

Australia • Brazil • Japan • Korea • Mexico • Singapore • Spain • United Kingdom • United States

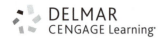

DELMAR
CENGAGE Learning·

Leading the Way, The Busy
Nurse's Guide to Supervision
in Long-Term Care, Third Edition
Karl Pillemer and Christine
Rheaume

Vice President, Career and
Computing: Dave Garza

Director of Learning Solutions:
Matthew Kane

Senior Acquisitions Editor:
Maureen Rosener

Managing Editor: Marah
Bellegarde

Product Manager: Samantha
L. Miller

Vice President, Career and
Professional Marketing: Jennifer
Ann Baker

Marketing Director: Wendy E.
Mapstone

Senior Marketing Manager:
Michele McTighe

Marketing Coordinator: Scott A.
Chrysler

Senior Production Director:
Wendy Troeger

Production Manager: Andrew
Crouth

Content Project Management:
PreMediaGlobal

Senior Art Director: Jack
Pendleton

Cover image: courtesy of
iStock.com

Library of Congress Control Number: 2011945102

ISBN-13: 978-1-133-13482-4

ISBN-10: 1-133-13482-3

Delmar
5 Maxwell Drive
Clifton Park, NY 12065-2919
USA

Cengage Learning is a leading provider of customized learning
solutions with office locations around the globe, including Singapore,
the United Kingdom, Australia, Mexico, Brazil, and Japan. Locate
your local office at: **international.cengage.com/region**

Cengage Learning products are represented in Canada by Nelson
Education, Ltd.

To learn more about Delmar, visit **www.cengage.com/delmar**

Purchase any of our products at your local college store or at our
preferred online store **www.cengagebrain.com**

Printed in the United States of America
1 2 3 4 5 6 7 16 15 14 13 12

TABLE OF CONTENTS

FOREWORD

Leading the Way is an important addition to the library of all nurse managers who want the very best from the people with whom they work. This book provides invaluable information about the tools for nursing leadership and key steps to building an effective team with high morale, productivity, and professionalism. It is not enough in this day and age to simply assign work and wait for the results. An effective supervisor understands that building a team that exudes trust and professionalism takes skill and energy. This book provides not only the essence of how those things are done but also practical examples that make the content easy to understand and apply. This third edition is thoroughly revised and updated, reflecting the progress in nursing management over the past decade. Nurses, long-term care facilities, and ultimately the residents will all benefit from those who read this material and take it to heart.

— Terry Fulmer, RN, PhD, FAAN,
Dean of the Bouvé College
of Health Sciences at Northeastern University

PREFACE

Expanded and revised, *Leading the Way: The Busy Nurse's Guide to Supervision in Long-Term Care, 3rd Edition* is intended to give nurses and supervisors-in-training the tools needed to experience and create success in any long-term care environment. This easy-to-read handbook applies proven methods from the latest research and covers everything from mentoring and motivating employees to dealing with job stress and ethical dilemmas. Succinct yet thorough, this new edition delivers the essentials of management and leadership, such as team building, communication, staff development, performance issues, and organization, all with a specific, long-term care focus. New discussions on strategies for staff development, effectively managing conflict, diffusing tension with humor, and achieving work/life balance make this guide even more useful for nursing professionals everywhere.

Conceptual Approach

Keep in mind that the book you are holding can be seen as a set of tools. What you do with these tools will help determine the experiences and successes in your long-term care environment. While we have provided a guide, it is up to you and your team to make it all come together. It is important to note that these tools can and should be adapted and modified by you so they work best for your staff and your facility.

By providing techniques for successful communication, strategies for staff development, and succinct tips for honing your leadership skills, the hope is that you will be the "champion" of your program—that, as the supervisor, you will continue your commitment to building an effective team with high morale, productivity, and professionalism.

Organization and Special Features

This guide has been designed to help you take on the challenges of being a supervisor and to make the transition from staff nurse to supervisor. It will present some of the challenges and expectations you need to be aware of, and offer advice from others who have been in your shoes.

Written in a straightforward, concise manner, each of the fifteen chapters begins with an overview of the topic being discussed. Tips and techniques for succeeding in your role as supervisor, provided through the use of checklists, quotes, and real-life examples, are followed in each chapter by a "Spotlight On" feature, which highlights the most vital information for easy reference. Each chapter is designed to be used independently or in conjunction with the others, so that the information you need is always at your fingertips.

New to This Edition

This third edition includes new material addressing effective collaboration to facilitate teamwork among staff at all levels. In a newly revised chapter, we tackle the important issue of stress reduction and suggest ways for supervisors to manage their own stress, and help employees to do the same. A new chapter on therapeutic humor in the workplace discusses the benefits of a good laugh to relieve stress, diffuse conflicts, and make the workplace more enjoyable.

A new chapter on Performance Management provides an overview of techniques to improve employee performance, conduct performance reviews, and implement corrective actions. We have also also included a chapter on staff development strategies, which reviews both formal and informal methods of training staff. Proven tips for making in-service sessions engaging and successful are offered. Finally, ethical dilemmas are common in long-term care nursing. This edition includes a new chapter that addresses the topic and equips readers with proven tactics for handling complex and sensitive situations.

ABOUT THE AUTHORS

Karl Pillemer

Karl Pillemer, PhD, is a Professor in the Department of Human Development at Cornell University and Professor of Gerontology in Medicine at the Weill Cornell Medical College. Dr. Pillemer has conducted research and developed practical programs to improve work life of nursing home staff. He has also consulted with long-term care providers around staffing issues. He has published five books and many scientific articles on nursing home staffing issues, including *Solving the Frontline Crisis in Long-Term Care.*

Christine Rheaume

Christine Rheaume, RN, is editor of educational materials for long-term care staff for Cengage Delmar Learning. A graduate of Massachusetts General Hospital School of Nursing, she has an extensive background in clinical nursing and in managed care environments. She is owner of Rheaume & Associates Legal Nurse Consulting Services.

Reviewers

Anna Ortigara, RN, MS, FAAN
Director of Communication and Outreach, THE GREEN HOUSE Project
Tinley Park, Illinois

Genevieve Gipson, RN, MEd, RNC
Director, National Network of Career Nursing Assistants
Norton, Ohio

Your Job As Supervisor

You have advanced in your career because of what you have achieved as an individual. As a nurse in long-term care, you have an additional challenge: to lead. Where once you might have been responsible solely for your own performance, you are now responsible for the performance of other caregivers.

Being a supervisor requires a nurse to think about things differently. As the leader of a caregiving team, you need to find ways to share your knowledge with others. And you must lead a group of caregivers with differing strengths and weaknesses. By discovering what motivates individual team members, you can tailor your approach as needed, and lead more effectively.

The Challenges of Today's Environment

The challenges of being a supervisor in today's fast-paced long-term care environment are many. Managing your staff and maintaining morale and professionalism under these circumstances require flexibility, effective planning, and insight into human nature.

As you reflect on your leadership responsibilities, it will be helpful to consider several important factors currently influencing the nursing home industry. One of these factors is the extreme staffing crisis nursing homes are facing today. Over the past five years, an already difficult staffing situation has reached a full-blown crisis. Most nursing homes across the country now identify their staffing problems as moderate or severe. The pool of applicants is shrinking, and the people who do apply often have limited job histories and little experience with the elderly and disabled.

Another important factor is the increasing impairment and complexity of the nursing home population. The emphasis on transferring elderly people from acute to long-term care settings as quickly as possible is partially due to the Medicare Prospective Payment System and from DRGs (Diagnosis Related Groups). This trend toward earlier discharge means that more residents remain acutely ill when they transfer to long-term care facilities.

One of the challenges associated with this trend is that nursing homes are now using more complicated technologies that were previously used only in hospitals. The burden of care for this increasingly impaired population often falls on nursing assistants. As a result, the job of frontline long-term care workers has changed dramatically. In just the past decade, nursing assistants' work has become much more complex, time-pressured, and stressful.

All of these factors will be important to you as you supervise and manage in today's reality. Remember that these challenges impact your staff significantly. To lead effectively, you must be flexible and realistic about your expectations. As a leader on nursing's frontline, you play a critical role in your facility by maintaining stability in an ever-changing environment.

Your Responsibilities as a Supervisor

Some of your job responsibilities are relatively easy to define but they can still be challenging in daily practice:

- Delegating responsibility for performance of specific tasks

- Providing concrete and reliable information about residents to their caregivers

- Listening to caregivers' observations about residents and responding as necessary

- Coaching and encouraging caregivers to constantly perform at their best

- Conducting performance evaluations of your team members

- Facilitating meetings, such as shift reports, intakes, and care-planning sessions

- Taking corrective actions and maintaining records of all necessary disciplinary measures

Other job responsibilities are not so easy to define. These include the following:

- Inspiring excellent caregiving

- Fostering a supportive, cooperative team spirit

- Teaching team members your facility's policies, procedures, and caregiving practices

- Serving as a link to other departments: PT/OT, Activities, Dietary, Social Work, Housekeeping, Administration, and Personnel

- Treating caregivers with the same respect and dignity they are asked to show to residents and their families

This book will help you take on the challenges of being a supervisor. However, don't feel that you must have all the answers; no one knows it all! And don't be afraid to ask questions. If a situation is new to you, someone out there has faced a similar challenge. Seek out that person, either within your facility or in the larger long-term care community. Remember that everyone likes to be asked for his or her opinion.

In your managerial role, you will be expected to:

- Be a visible and effective leader to the entire team

- Address problems immediately—either by yourself or with the help of your supervisor or administrator—and document them

- Plan your day, week, and month to meet your team's caregiving objectives

- Finish your work and paperwork before you leave for the day

- Take action whenever you see someone who is in trouble or causing problems—whether or not he or she is on your team

- Maintain the confidentiality of information given to you by your facility's administration and sharing confidential information about caregivers only with the appropriate administrative staff (e.g., personnel or human resources)

The job of a supervisor can be challenging. You need to earn the confidence and trust of your team, encourage them to exceed their own expectations, and monitor the performance of individuals and the team as a whole.

This book will help you make the transition from thinking of yourself as a staff nurse to thinking of yourself as a supervisor who must sometimes get the job done by managing others. It will present some of the challenges and expectations you may encounter in this role. Think of it as advice from others who have been in your shoes.

CHAPTER 1

What Is Leadership?

"You can only lead others where you yourself are willing to go."
—Lachlan McLean

What is a leader? Is a leader born or made? Is leadership a function of one's character? Or is it a set of skills that can be taught? Webster's Dictionary defines leadership as guidance, direction, or "showing the way." Stephen Covey, a renowned leadership expert and author, tells us that we "lead people and manage things." Leadership is not an inborn trait, but instead it is a series of acquired skills. Research into the dynamics of leadership suggests that most people have the potential to become leaders in the right circumstances and with attention to strengthening their interpersonal skills. With the knowledge and desire to show the way, a person can be a leader.

What Your Role Means

Being given a leadership role means that your facility's administration has confidence in your character and abilities. You have been given the authority to make decisions about how direct care will be provided by the caregivers you supervise. Ultimately, you are accountable for the success of your team, as measured by resident well-being, quality improvement scales, and surveys.

Your leadership role requires you to begin thinking in different ways that will ultimately lead to the delivery of higher quality care to residents. You will have to:

- create a vision and sense of community
- foster commitment rather than compliance
- integrate diverse views
- help others express their opinions
- facilitate, energize, and sustain those who work for you

Some people think that only certain personality types— outgoing or extroverted people, for example—make good leaders. This is not true. Each successful leader has a unique style; however, they share three key characteristics—vision, planning, and flexibility—that can be learned and practiced by people with all sorts of personalities.

1. Vision

Having vision means not only knowing what your destination or goal is, but having the desire, motivation, and skills to get there. When setting goals for your caregiving team, remember to be specific. For example, quality care is not a specific goal. Quality care is an ideal, a core value to keep in mind at all times. A goal is something different. Once it is reached, a goal that is modest, achievable, and stated in positive terms will energize a team for greater challenges.

On the other hand, choosing a goal that cannot be reached will eventually leave your team demoralized and weakened. Think of those all-or-nothing New Year's resolutions we make each year. How many of them do we accomplish? To be realistic, a team's goal should probably contain the words *to improve* or *to better*. For example, "to improve participation in in-service programs" is a better goal than "to ensure perfect attendance" at in-services. It is always easier to stay focused on a goal that is stated positively. For example, to "improve attendance" is more motivating than to "reduce absenteeism."

Having a vision is not sufficient by itself, even if you have turned that vision into specific goals. You must be able to communicate it—in your own style—to the other members of the caregiving team, and provide encouragement when the team loses energy or focus, reminding team members of the goal.

The best leaders lead by example. By encouraging, complimenting, and appreciating team members, the leader shows the way, not only to the goal but also to better teamwork.

Let's look at a specific example of leadership in long-term care.

Terry, a nurse manager, is in charge of a unit where many of the residents suffer from dementia and often act out in an aggressive manner, sometimes injuring the CNAs. She has noticed that her staff are angry and bewildered by this situation because they lack the knowledge necessary to understand the causes of aggressive behaviors. Terry first coordinates an effort with the medical and nursing staff to rule out an underlying medical cause of the residents' behavior, such as pain or medication side effect. She then discusses the problem of resident aggression with the director of nursing, social worker, and administrator. She shares many examples from her experience on the unit and together they decide that an in-service training needs to be developed on injury prevention and dementia care.

In this example, Terry uses her experience and communication skills to share her **individual vision** with the administrative team, and partners with them in a group **vision** for solving the problem.

2. Planning

Planning is the companion to vision; it is the way your team achieves its goals. Before starting a new activity, a supervisor should consider not only what objectives must be achieved but also how to monitor progress toward those objectives. Some jobs are too large or complex for one person. As a supervisor, you must determine which caregivers work best together, and assign them accordingly. You may have to plan for certain procedures to be performed by personnel across shifts. It is your responsibility to translate your team's goals into day-to-day activities, turning the vision into tangible results.

*The next step in Terry's process is to provide her input into the **planning** process. She works with facility staff to clearly identify the goals of the in-service and develop measurable objectives. Terry reinforces the new information from the in-service training with the CNAs on her unit in day-to-day practice. She observes and coaches the CNAs, instructing them in ways to avoid injury. She notices that Frank, one of the more experienced nursing assistants, has a natural, skillful way of protecting himself* *from aggressive behavior from the residents. Terry asks Frank to share his approach with others at a staff meeting. Before and after the in-service, Terry carefully documents the number of times residents on the unit injure CNAs. She communicates successes to the staff and celebrates their improved outcomes.*

3. Flexibility

Handling the unexpected is a key part of supervising any group. Schedules always change, often in ways that could stand in the way of meeting your goals. A supervisor must be able to make last-minute changes, large and small, in the plan. In a nursing facility, staff turnover, changing acuity levels of residents, and new admissions all contribute to rapid change. You will often have to make on-the-spot decisions to re-deploy staff, or shift the team's emphasis from one area of caregiving to another. For example, if three out of twelve nursing assistants call in sick with the flu, you must reassign the remaining members of your team and draw on temporary help who may not be familiar with the residents.

Terry is seeing measurable results in efforts to prevent CNA injuries on her unit. One day, however, she falls and breaks her leg, and is unable to work for the next two months. When Terry returns to work, most of the CNAs are new, and lack injury prevention knowledge and skills. Although she feels discouraged, she discusses the situation with the director of nursing, social worker, and administrator, and they schedule another injury prevention in-service. Together, they decide to repeat the in-service as often as needed to make it accessible to new staff. Terry realizes that she has to be persistent and flexible in her ongoing efforts to provide guidance and to coach staff in the skills necessary to protect themselves.

Project Planning Process

1. Visualize and state the goals of this project.
- List the problems that this project will solve.
- Identify how residents and/or staff will benefit.

2. Get support and official approval from your supervisor and others necessary to make it happen.
- Collect data and estimate potential benefits.

3. List all the resources you will need.
- Estimate costs.
- Estimate how many and what types of staff support will be needed.

4. Develop a detailed project plan.
- List steps (separate activities).
- Designate who will do which steps.
- Set deadlines by which each step must be completed.

5. Conduct project.
- Document participation.

6. Evaluate progress.
- Were the project goals achieved?
- What evidence can you show that the goals were met?
- Communicate outcome and progress to staff.

CHAPTER 2

Building an Effective Team

"Coming together is a beginning; keeping together is progress; working together is success."
—*Henry Ford*

As anyone who has played on an athletic team knows, working on a team reinforces the realization that others are depending on us. Teams are a natural choice for giving good care; they underscore the relationships between everyone in the nursing facility, improve results, and make the work easier. Just as a sports team wins games by working together, a caregiving team wins by working together to provide the care residents deserve and their families expect. It isn't always easy, but working as a team offers many advantages.

Effective Caregiving Teams

Effective caregiving teams are organized around three central principles: trust, balance, and professionalism. These principles have powerful implications in your day-to-day work as a supervisor.

1. Trust

Communicating your trust in the team empowers them to get the job done. By ensuring adequate training, and keeping the team focused on their common goals, you know you can trust each member to perform his or her job well.

2. Balance

When you work in teams, the strengths and weaknesses of individual team members balance one another, and the entire group is stronger as a result. Balance also applies to our work and outside-of-work responsibilities. As a supervisor, you may need to help your team members learn to juggle their work and family responsibilities. Leadership means keeping "the big picture" in mind and guiding staff toward shared goals.

3. Professionalism

Professionalism includes not only how we relate to residents and their families but also how we treat one another. As the leader, you set the tone for your team's professionalism by treating your team members with respect.

In today's long-term care environment, facilities must be able to change as conditions demand. The tendency toward higher acuity of long-term care residents, medical advances, and changes in reimbursement structures are only a few of the many factors that make the world of long-term care less stable than it used to be. The diverse experience and skills of all caregivers, from the newest staff members to the most seasoned veterans, are valuable in meeting these new challenges as they arise. Helping your team work together allows them to achieve their full potential, provides opportunities for mutual learning, and reduces the risk of burnout.

The Four Styles of Team Participation

Experts have identified four styles of team participation.* Your caregiving team is likely to include people with differing styles. The job of a supervisor is to elicit the best performance from each team member. Recognizing and understanding the different styles of team participation will help you to to better moderate discussions, resolve conflicts, and encourage team members to use their strengths to the fullest. This insight will also help you recognize where team members might need more coaching.

The four styles are the following:

1. **The Contributor** enjoys providing the team with good information or new methods of working. This team member is dependable, organized, and detail-focused but might not see the larger picture. When working with this person, provide complete and detailed information, as the Contributor tends to take detailed and specific information most seriously. You may need to help the Contributor understand the big picture by providing the background and reasoning that underlies a project or task.

---

* Parker, G.M. (2008) Team Players and Teamwork: New Strategies for the Competitive Enterprise, Second Edition. San Francisco, CA: John Wiley and Sons.

2. **The Collaborator** is flexible, imaginative, and goal-directed. The Collaborator is open to new ideas but sometimes fails to give enough attention to basic tasks. With a Collaborator, you will find a partner to help implement new projects, but you may need to remind this team member to focus on the specific, incremental tasks involved.

3. **The Communicator** helps facilitate discussion, build consensus, and resolve conflict. The Communicator may not like to confront others and sometimes may get caught up in a process rather than focusing on results. The Communicator can be one of your greatest assets if you remind him or her of expected results, and enlist this person in building enthusiasm for a project among other team members.

4. **The Challenger** encourages the team to take risks. This team member is outspoken, principled, and adventurous but sometimes can try to push the team too far. To work with a Challenger, you'll need to rein in some of the person's riskier ideas and help him or her focus more realistically on the project goals.

Keep in mind that some of your team members may prefer to work on their own. It is important to communicate that working on a team doesn't have to mean giving up autonomy and job satisfaction. These people often become the most enthusiastic members of the team when they realize that their contributions are valued.

Part of your job is to facilitate the exchange of ideas and information. You can do this by asking individuals to share their expertise with the group. You might also suggest that someone lead a team project such as planning for National Nursing Assistants Week, managing resident laundry, or creating a fair and equitable "float list." Another way to foster this kind of communication is to hold regular team meetings during which you encourage discussion of caregiving problems from a variety of perspectives.

People tend to work best in teams because this allows everyone to contribute experience and skills to help solve problems and, often, to have some fun while doing so. Experienced caregivers can still learn from the fresh perspective of newcomers, while new caregivers can become more adept by working with and observing experienced staff. If your facility has adopted consistent assignment, a model in which residents receive care from the same caregivers each day, you may be even more successful in building a strong, cohesive team.

Building your team on the principles of trust, balance, and professionalism will encourage each member to put forth his or her best effort. Understanding the four styles of participation will help you to make the most of each person's contribution. Once you have your team in place, its effectiveness depends largely on communication, the topic of the next chapter.

Teamwork—A Parable

There is a story about a man who was invited to take a tour of heaven and hell. First his guide led him to a room where a group of people sat around a circular table. Each had one arm tied behind his back. The other arm was in a straight, rigid cast, and each person held a long-handled spoon in that hand.

A steaming bowl of a delicious-smelling stew sat in the middle of the table, but none of the people could eat from it because none could bend his elbow. The people were terribly thin and sickly. They suffered greatly, not only from hunger but also from the great frustration of having the stew so close by.

"This is hell," said the guide.

"I can see that," said the tourist.

Then the guide opened another door. Another group of people were seated around the same kind of table, one arm tied behind their backs, the other arm in a straight cast with a long-handled spoon in that hand. The same bowl of stew sat in the middle of the table. But these people were happy, and healthy-looking. As the tourist watched, one of the people dipped his spoon in the stew and reached it across the table to feed another. Over and over again as he watched, the people helped one another taste the delicious stew.

"And this," said the guide, "is heaven."

CHAPTER 3

Communication: The Secret of Successful Supervision

"Seek first to understand, then to be understood."
—*St. Francis of Assisi*

In your position as a supervisor, how well you communicate with your team members, both verbally and nonverbally, influences their job satisfaction. For example, if you are too critical without providing positive feedback to a particular team member, that team member's morale may suffer. He or she may even begin to dread coming to work. The messages you send should convey that you value the team members' strengths and can help them, in a respectful and constructive manner, to work on their weak areas.

Listening Skills

Many times, people who are thought of as good communicators are, in reality, good listeners. As a clinician, you learned to listen attentively to residents to discover their needs and concerns. By satisfying those needs, you were able to provide quality care. In the same way, listening to your team members' needs and concerns helps you to spot problems early and work toward resolving them.

Remember, most people love to talk about themselves. As individuals speak to you about their own feelings and experiences, you are learning how their perceptions, attitudes, and feelings relate to the larger group.

Good listening skills include the following:

• Allowing the other person to talk without interrupting.

• Providing nonverbal cues—such as nodding your head, saying "I see"—that demonstrate you understand what the other person is saying.

• Maintaining eye contact.

• Asking open-ended questions (ones that require more than a "yes" or "no" answer).

• Summarizing or recapping the problem so that the other person knows you heard and understood.

By listening, you learn what motivates your team—pride in a job well done, an expression of appreciation from a resident or family member, recognition, awards, the opportunity for advancement. You can then use those motivations to reinforce core values and best practices. Good listening skills also help you tune into the concerns and anxieties of individual team members and become aware of any problems in their personal lives that may be preventing them from doing a good job. You may also learn more about achievements that can be celebrated and about the group's morale. Listening actively will give you information that helps you do your job better and will help your team provide the highest quality care.

Using "I" Messages

Active listening is only one part of good communication. You also need to know how to deliver your own messages effectively. Use of "I" messages is a good method for saying what you mean in a clear and respectful manner. Sometimes you will understand a person's perspective but not agree with it. When this happens, you need to let that person know how you feel, show that you understand how he or she feels, and then present a compromise or solution to the problem. Practice using the model on the following page until you become comfortable with it. Your interactions with your staff will be greatly enhanced.

Receiving Criticism

It is almost certain that you'll hear negative comments about you or your facility in your role as a supervisor. Although maintaining a thick skin when hearing (or overhearing) criticism is difficult, there are important reasons for ignoring comments that are not offered in the spirit of helpfulness. Reacting to undue criticism only escalates the situation and places it on a personal level. By refusing to react to hostile remarks, you also enhance your image of objectivity and professionalism.

Remember that not all unwelcome comments are inappropriate. Keep an open mind when staff members share their frustrations, and listen for the underlying issue. Your willingness to hear and consider alternative viewpoints demonstrates your strength as a leader.

THE "I" MESSAGE

A. *When _____ happens,*

B. *I feel _____,*

C. *because _____.*

D. *I would like _____ to happen.*

Begin with a brief description of what's on your mind.

When you arrive late for work . . .

Then describe how you feel about it.

I feel worried . . .

And why you feel that way.

. . . because residents don't get the morning care they need.

If you know what you want to have happen, say so.

I would like to find a way to work with you so you arrive on time for all of your shifts.

Then, use your best listening skills to hear what the other person tells you about the situation. You will learn something valuable, and the other person will feel respected. Notice that there is no judgment expressed in this message.

This type of communication may feel somewhat unnatural at first, but you will be surprised at how well it can work. Good listening skills and "I" messages are especially helpful in tough situations when you want to get your message across without blaming.

However, should you ever directly hear criticism that seems threatening to you or any other person in the facility, report it immediately to your administrator.

Providing Feedback

To maintain the trust of your team members, it is important that you give them plenty of honest, constructive feedback. Even when your feedback is critical of a team member's performance, phrasing it in a positive, useful way makes it more likely that the person will be motivated to improve his or her performance.

For example, rather than telling a member of your staff, "You are feeding Mrs. Smith all wrong," try phrasing your response in terms of past successes: "I can see that you have been trying to improve your feeding technique. Let me demonstrate a method that I think you will find works better."

Constructive feedback helps a person discover his or her own capabilities and suggests a course of action for reaching goals. When you have to recommend corrective action—the process of documenting a failure to follow the facility's policies and procedures—your team members will need support and encouragement to make positive behavior changes.

SPOTLIGHT ON . . .

Structured Communication Tips

1. Schedule regular staff meetings.

Meetings can serve two purposes. First, they can get people together to solve a problem or to discuss a critical topic. Second, they can keep people informed of what is going on in the workplace. Regularly scheduled meetings can save time and improve communication by proactively addressing work challenges.

2. Maintain a staff suggestion box.

A staff suggestion box can enhance communication by giving people the chance to express their opinions about a wide variety of work-related issues. Place a box with an inexpensive lock (to which you have the key) in an accessible area for workers, and supply paper and a pen. Make sure that the box is in a convenient yet discreet location. Check the box at least once a week, and discuss these suggestions in your regularly scheduled staff meetings.

3. Have change-of-shift reporting sessions.

It's extremely useful to bring together the caregivers who are just getting off work with those who are just coming on. Even five minutes with both groups can help to ensure continuity of care. The change-of-shift reporting session is an ideal time to highlight the individual needs of a particular resident and helps the incoming shift to anticipate problems. This time is also useful for caregivers on different shifts to get to know each other better. However, the primary focus of these meetings should be on residents and their care needs, and not on socialization.

4. Recognize successful communications.

Make it a practice to recognize and celebrate your staff for communicating effectively. You might offer a regular "Communicator of the Month" recognition for someone who shares a good suggestion or important information about a resident.

CHAPTER 4

Setting an Example: Teaching and Mentoring

"Better than a thousand days of diligent study is one day with a great teacher."
—*Japanese Proverb*

In becoming a supervisor, you have already demonstrated that you have a good grasp of the best caregiving practices. A key part of your job is to mentor new caregivers and set an example for all members of your team, so that they can continue to learn and grow professionally. You have come to this point in your career with many rich experiences as a nursing professional. Your knowledge and skills will enhance the ability of your staff to provide high-quality care for the residents in your facility. The best way of passing on the benefits of your experiences, knowledge, and skills is through the teaching and mentoring role.

Inspiring Excellence

People can be encouraged to improved levels of performance by the example you set. The daily demands of your job can make it difficult to think about the example you're setting, but nothing speaks more clearly to the members of your team. From time to time, try to step back from the hustle to ask yourself if you're being the best role model you can be. Here are some questions you might want to consider:

- Am I being patient in explaining new concepts to team members?

- Do I answer each question as if it were the first time I'd heard it?

- Am I pleasant when answering questions?

- Do I provide positive feedback as well as feedback on the need for improvement?

- Do I bring enthusiasm and commitment to my work?

- Do I clearly communicate my expectations?

- Do I provide my team members with the support, encouragement, and training they need to do their jobs well?

- Am I trustworthy when given personal and confidential information?

Answering "yes" to these questions will not guarantee that you'll have a committed, dependable, and expert caregiving team—but it will set the stage for developing one. Your team members will know that they can seek your advice without being criticized for what they don't know. They will see you as a positive and enthusiastic role model. Your supervisory interactions will be easier, and the care your team provides will continually improve.

Learning Styles

When working with your team, keep in mind that your own style of learning will not work for everyone. For example, you may prefer learning a new skill by reading instructions, while others may learn better by watching a procedure or by doing it themselves with coaching and advice. By the time we reach adulthood, we have developed certain ways of learning that work best for us.

Most adults use a combination of learning styles, one of the following styles will be most comfortable:

- The **visual learner** might say, "Show me. I'll watch. Then I'll know how."

- The **auditory learner** prefers to hear instructions: "If you explain it to me clearly, then I'll know how to do it."

- The **cognitive** or **thinking learner** might say, "Give me written directions. Let me study it, and I'll learn it."

- The **kinesthetic** or **doing** learner prefers trial and error: "Just let me do it over until I get it right. Then I'll know it."

It is important to know your preferred learning style. As teacher or coach, it's best not to rely solely on your own learning style to teach others. Try to identify the preferred learning style of each member of your staff by asking them to recall a successful learning experience. Here are some examples of successful learning experiences:

- *Tanisha might remember learning how to ride a bike by watching others (visual learner).*

- *Terry might remember learning to make a pizza by listening to a description of how to do it (auditory learner).*

- *Sue might remember learning how to apply eye makeup by reading a magazine description on the proper technique (cognitive or thinking learner).*

- *Tony might remember how he learned to dance by trying over and over to perfect the right moves (kinesthetic or doing learner).*

These examples will provide you with important clues about how each staff member learns best. As a coach, you will be more successful if you try to appeal to that person's learning style.

Another facet of mentoring is acting as a role model. Treating everyone with respect and in a pleasant manner will inspire your team members to show respect for each other. The way you interact with your supervisor and peers will also set an example for the way your team members interact with you.

As a leader, it is important to remember that your staff are constantly observing you and how you treat others. Modeling respectful behavior provides your staff with a powerful tool for maintaining respectful interactions with residents, visitors, and one another.

As a nurse manager, you will be called on to demonstrate and teach skills to the CNAs. Try to become aware of their learning styles as well as your own. The following guidelines can help you perform these teaching tasks with skill and expertise.

Guidelines for Successful Teaching Practice

1. **Prepare** learners by making sure that they know the learning goals.

2. **Provide** a safe, comfortable environment so that staff can engage in an uninterrupted learning experience.

3. **Demonstrate** the skill or skills in a calm, orderly way. If there are several steps, demonstrate each one clearly.

4. Allow your staff to **practice** the skill immediately after it is demonstrated.

5. **Observe** staff members while they practice the skill, then give concrete feedback, coaching until they perform the task successfully. During the next week, observe them whenever possible to note their progress.

CHAPTER 5

Strategies for Staff Development

"Life is like a band. We need not all play the same part, but we must all play in harmony."
—*(unknown author)*

Long-term care staff at all levels must be competent in their roles, not only to satisfy regulatory requirements but most importantly to provide excellent care to residents. Your job as supervisor is to encourage your staff to strive for this goal by offering stimulating learning opportunities. You can accomplish this by providing meaningful and relevant learning activities that are cost-effective for your organization.

Key Principles

An important first step in designing a staff development plan is to assess the educational needs of those who will take part in it. Involving employees in this process increases their commitment and interest and provides an opportunity to align the training program with the goals and mission of the facility.

Here are some important principles to remember:

- Evaluate competency based on employee performance evaluations and family/resident satisfaction surveys. Ask: What does your staff need to know?

- Know your audience. Prepare handouts and other materials at the appropriate level for the target staff.

- Understand your state's regulatory requirements for covering specific topics at a designated frequency for certain groups of employees such as nursing assistants.

- Collect self-assessment data from staff to determine their perceived gaps in knowledge or competency.

- Ask staff to suggest topics of interest to them.

Strategy and Delivery

A good staff development plan is an ongoing, dynamic process that includes a mix of formal and informal in-service sessions. Learning goals must be realistic and stated clearly up front, along with a timeframe for attaining these objectives. A written outline of key points to be covered provides participants with a logical "road map" to follow during the training session, and can be a valuable tool for later review.

Brief, on-the-spot in-services conducted on the unit or at the bedside can be effective because they actively engage the learner. This approach works especially well for topics with a hands-on component, such as a nursing procedure review or to teach the proper use of equipment.

Electronic media including CD-ROM, DVD, and Internet resources offer a wide array of educational material in the field of geriatric nursing and other topics relevant to long-term care. Although some of these options can come with a hefty price tag, remember that they can be used multiple times, or at least until the material becomes outdated. Also, factor in the ability to offer the same high-quality material to all shifts, and the convenience of self-study when considering purchase value. However, avoid relying exclusively on electronic resources as a substitute for personalized teaching opportunities. Be available to staff for questions and feedback related to the educational materials provided.

Staff development doesn't have to be expensive. When planning in-service presentations, try to use expertise that already exists within your own nursing staff and other departments in your organization. Consulting physicians, pharmacists, therapists, and department heads are often happy to present on a topic relevant to their area. Bringing in an outside speaker—a representative from a local organization, college, referring hospital, or vendor—can also be stimulating for the staff and enhance the relationship between the facility and the community.

Considerations for Adult Learners

Many adults are intimidated by the "student" role, whether in a formal classroom or an informal setting. A comfortable environment, supportive atmosphere, and open dialogue between instructors and participants help to facilitate learning by keeping stress to a minimum.

Teaching formats that actively engage the student have a much better chance of success. For example, involving students in a pre-presentation activity that informally tests their knowledge of the subject piques their interest in the subject. Be creative in finding ways to liven up presentations. We too often follow the "sage on a stage" lecture model. Remember that the use of more than one sense enhances adult learning. Judicious use of props, quizzes, jokes, or "brain teasers" can break the ice and make the session and its content more memorable.

Educational experts tell us that adults respond best when learning is:

- Participatory/hands-on

- Student-centered

- Relevant to "real life" situations

- Respectful of the learner's expertise

- Motivated both externally and internally

The timing of educational programs is important. Expecting employees to attend mandatory in-service sessions on their off-duty time can be unrealistic. Providing training opportunities on work time when possible—and on all shifts—demonstrates the organization's commitment to its staff and respect for their need for personal time away from work. Many facilities find that scheduling training programs around the time of shift changes can allow more staff to attend. Presenting more complex topics in a series of several short modules not only maximizes learning potential but also has less impact on staffing.

Evaluating Results

Evaluating the staff development presentation or activity brings us full circle, back to the stated goals of the training session. How well did the session meet these goals? The following four levels of evaluation will help you to decide:

Participant Reaction: Was the information relevant to their work? Was it presented at an appropriate level?

Evaluate With: participant questionnaire

This means more than requiring employees to turn in a hastily filled-in form at the end of a training session. It involves initiating and maintaining an ongoing dialogue with the staff about their learning needs and how well you are addressing them. Nurse leaders have an opportunity to motivate employees to learn by being receptive to constructive criticism and welcoming their input.

New Skills: Does the staff possess new knowledge/skills as a result of the presentation?

Evaluate With: post-presentation quiz

For some adult learners, the prospect of "test taking" resurrects old fears related to previous school experiences. You can help to set the stage for success by acknowledging these feelings, which can otherwise impede learning and the flow of information between instructor and student.

Behavior Change: Did the presentation result in staff behavior change related to the stated goal?

Evaluate With: periodic employee performance evaluation

Systemwide Effect: Is there a measurable impact on quality of care, cost effectiveness, error rate?

Evaluate With: data collection and analysis

The overarching goal of staff development is to provide competent care to residents, to enhance their life quality, and to meet regulatory requirements. As a leader in this effort, you can play a big part in fostering the professional growth of every member of your team.

CHAPTER 6

Documentation

"If you have knowledge, let others light their candles with it."
—*Margaret Fuller*

Nurse managers play an important role in influencing the quality of documentation on their units. As the health care system becomes more complex, the emphasis on documentation increases. There are many reasons for this shift, including regulatory changes, accreditation, and legal and financial factors. Most residents in long-term care facilities are vulnerable, and their health status can change rapidly. Close observation and prompt communication of their changing needs can help prevent a serious decline in health and improve their life quality. Accurate documentation of the care that is given to a resident also can be an important factor in defending the facility in the event of a lawsuit.

As a supervisor, it is your role not only to know how to document clearly but also to make sure that nursing assistants are able to do the same. CNAs need to know how to document and why it is critically important that they do so accurately and regularly.

Teaching CNAs to Document

If staff members see documentation as a way of ensuring the well-being of residents, they are more likely to maintain good documentation habits. CNAs need to understand the value of their contribution to documentation. The Medicare Prospective Payment System (PPS) acknowledges the importance of this work and values the nursing assistant's firsthand knowledge of each resident. Nurse managers must let CNAs know that their documentation is an essential part of providing good care.

The current PPS system makes every staff person accountable, not only for the quality of care a resident receives but also for the quality of the communication on which the care planning process rests. Ultimately the nurse manager is responsible for delegating documentation tasks to nursing assistants and for maintaining the ongoing quality of the documentation practice.

Be aware of the learning styles of your staff as you teach them the documentation process. Some nursing assistants will understand the process best if you demonstrate it, others when you describe it, and others when they read directions. Chances are that you will need to present the process in different ways and coach your staff regularly to make sure that they are keeping accurate and timely records.

MDS = BETTER Care

The Minimum Data Set (MDS) is the record of care for each resident. It must be based on accurate information about the actual care provided. Generally speaking, a licensed nurse will be responsible for completing the MDS based on professional nursing assessment of the resident. As integral members of the care team, CNAs have valuable information to share about individual residents. Each organization has its own policies regarding how these observations are recorded. Some facilities make it a practice to interview CNAs about the residents. Others train CNAs to record the care they give on special forms or checklists (and, increasingly, electronically). You will need to tailor your approach to supporting the documentation process based on your facility's established policies and procedures.

Remember that the key to good documentation practice is to teach your staff to observe and record the needs of the residents and their care. When documenting this care, **BETTER** is a helpful memory aid for reminding nursing assistants to focus on the following Activities of Daily Living (ADLs). Let's take a look at each of these areas of **BETTER** care.

Bed Mobility

How does the resident move to and from a lying position? Turn from side to side? Position his body while in bed? How much assistance, if any, does the resident require? This is also a good time to observe the condition of the resident's skin, and note any signs of pain.

Eating

How much help does the resident need at mealtime? Does the resident require set-up help? Assistance with feeding? Does the resident require your undivided attention for the course of the meal? How well is the resident eating? Have you learned some additional information about his or her preferences? This is also a good time to observe and record any changes in the resident's appetite.

Transfer

How does the resident move from one surface to another, from wheelchair to bed, for example? How much assistance does the resident need?

Toileting

Does the resident use a toilet or bedpan on his or her own or with help? Does the resident require assistance during this transfer? Can the resident manage his or her own ostomy or catheter? Is there a scheduled toileting plan in place, such as prompted voiding or habit training?

Emotional/Behavioral Status

Look for changes in the resident's mood and behavior. Has the resident lost interest in activities? Does he or she seem anxious, depressed, or angry or fearful? Is the resident having trouble sleeping? (These can be the first symptoms of infection.) Has the resident refused care or expressed feelings of despair, such as "Nothing matters anymore" or "Nobody cares about me"? Does the resident wander or exhibit socially inappropriate behaviors such as public nudity, smearing food or feces, hitting, biting, or other inappropriate touching?

Be sure to note positive changes, too. Statements such as "I'm going to beat this illness!" or "I'm really looking forward to getting my hair done" may be signs that a resident's care plan is working well, that medication is helping, or that medical status is improving. You can note the resident's emotional and behavioral status while assisting with ADLs and throughout the day.

Restorative Care

In many nursing homes, CNAs perform certain kinds of restorative care under the guidance of the PT/OT department. Restorative care can be Range of Motion (ROM) or any other program of exercise or therapeutic activity such as walking, training with light weights, or massage.

If we want to provide more than just basic physical care (and of course we do!) we should delve even deeper. How does the resident feel about being in this facility? What are this individual's hopes and dreams? The Minimum Data Set (MDS) is a tool that helps the care team gather necessary information in a standardized way, ensuring that no aspect of the nursing home residents' needs is overlooked.

Communicating about Documentation

The communication skills discussed earlier in this book can help you support the documentation process. As you observe your staff's documentation efforts, it is important to provide honest, constructive feedback. Even when the feedback is critical of performance, phrasing it in a positive, useful way makes it more effective.

For example, rather than saying, "Your documentation is sloppy," try phrasing your response in terms of past successes: "You have excellent observation skills, but often you don't take credit for all that you do. Let's work together on a plan to improve your written documentation." This feedback reinforces the nursing assistant's efforts and fosters a positive attitude about continuing to improve.

Tips for Maintaining Good Documentation Practice

Be a good role model.

- As a manager, practice good documentation habits.
- Model a high standard for the staff.

Make sure CNAs know why they're documenting.

- Emphasize the benefits for residents.
- Clarify liability and regulatory issues.

Teach CNAs to document.

- Be aware of staff learning styles.
- Present information in multiple ways.
- Make sure that staff members know medical terminology and acceptable abbreviations.
- Emphasize the importance of legible writing.

Communicate the importance of good practice.

- Give positive feedback when appropriate.
- Encourage efforts to improve.

Use a team approach.

- Make sure nursing assistants know that they are essential members of the team.
- Clarify roles of supervisor and nursing assistants in the documentation process.

Recognize CNAs for documenting well.

- Informal recognition: Make positive comments on daily practice when appropriate.

- Formal recognition: Offer awards for successful documentation.

CHAPTER 7

Managing and Organizing for Success

"Lost time is never found again."
—*Benjamin Franklin*

Good organizational skills are a valuable asset when it comes to managing frontline staff. However, you don't have to be a "naturally" well-organized person to successfully manage your team. These skills can be learned and continuously honed as you discover your own personal management style. Planning, setting goals, and managing your time effectively can lead you to success as a leader in your facility.

Establishing Performance Goals

What is a goal? A goal is an objective that you and your team want to reach. On an athletic team, the goal is clear: to win games. In health care, caregiving excellence is the ultimate goal. However, it is necessary to define the elements of excellent care and to develop goals that allow the team to measure its success.

The two steps of goal setting are (1) choosing an objective and (2) motivating the team to reach the objective. Take your time when identifying objectives, because unreachable goals can be a source of frustration for a team.

Goals should be:

- **specific**—be as clear and exact as you can about the goal.

- **measurable**—there should be a way to determine whether or not you've reached the goal.

- **realistic**—the goal should take into account your resources as well as the team's strengths and weaknesses.

- **attainable**—set your sights high, but not too high; make sure it's a goal you can reach.

Remember, goals need to be carefully thought out and designed to maximize team spirit. If goals become unattainable or unrealistic, change them. If a goal does not work out the way you anticipate, engage the team in devising a more reasonable target.

Tips for Staying Organized

As you work on goals, organizational skills are your secret weapon. These tips will help you to "bring order to chaos."

1. Handle a piece of paper (or an e-mail) only once: File it, send it on to someone else, or discard it.

2. Keep a notebook handy to capture ideas and tasks that you want to remember.

3. Keep a calendar with meeting appointments, schedules, and other time-related information.

4. Set up a filing system that's easy to use and maintain.

5. Have a place for everything, and return things to their place immediately after you've used them.

Managing Time

When you are overrun with work at your job, the last thing you want to do is stop moving. Yet this actually *is* the time to stop for a moment to focus on setting priorities and delegating. These two powerful techniques—prioritizing and delegating—will help you manage your time more effectively and accomplish what's really necessary. Make a list of all the things that need to be done and highlight the most important tasks. These take special precedence. Look at the list again. Can you delegate any of these tasks to someone else? Once you have decided what has to be done and what has to be done by you, then you can continue working. Time that you take now for focusing, prioritizing, and delegating will save you time in the long run.

Prioritization

Prioritization is a process of listing tasks or actions in order of the most to the least important. Prioritizing lets you focus on the most essential tasks when you are pressed for time. It also allows you to schedule non-urgent tasks for times when you know you won't be so busy. As a leader, you need to be aware of the long-range plans and overarching goals of your area. Thinking about the "bigger picture" will help you to coordinate your team's efforts toward these larger goals.

Delegating

Delegating is assigning appropriate tasks to workers rather than doing every task yourself. Many supervisors feel that "if you want to get something done around here you have to do it yourself." Unfortunately, this belief is misguided and unproductive. Giving work to others helps you manage your time and meet your long-range goals. It also gives important and exciting tasks to other workers and demonstrates faith in your team members.

Time Management Strategies that Really Work

- **Make to-do lists.** Take time to think about and write down a brief list of what needs to be done.

- **Set goals.** Write down your goals and place them where you can easily see them throughout the day.

- **Identify your individual work style.** Are you a "multitasker," or do you work better tackling one task at a time?

- **Maximize your most productive times.** Be aware of your internal clock and at what hours you are at your best. Schedule your day according to this internal clock and use this time for your most involved or difficult tasks.

- **Stay focused.** Everyone wants to be nice, but don't accept tasks that you don't have the time to complete. Avoid spreading yourself and your time too thin.

- **Don't waste time.** There is a fine line between walking around and making yourself available to staff, and wasting time outright. You must find this balance—especially if you find yourself avoiding tasks.

- **Shield yourself from distractions.** Set aside time each day to be undisturbed except for emergencies, so that complex tasks receive the attention they need.

CHAPTER 8

Recognition Equals High Morale

"If the only prayer you say in life is 'thank you,' that would suffice."
—*Meister Eckhart*

One of your most important challenges is motivating the nursing assistants you supervise. Today's nursing assistants often feel unrecognized and underappreciated. In focus groups and surveys, nursing assistants often say things like: "We always hear right away when we've done something wrong, but we never hear when we do something right!"

Decades of studies about how people learn and how they change their behavior have taught us one simple truth: Rewards are much more effective than punishment and criticism in motivating people to improve their performance.

It's actually quite simple: Consistent recognition of accomplishments leads to higher staff retention rates. This concept is especially relevant for supervisors in nursing home settings. Research has shown that nursing assistants—the majority of staff you supervise—feel disempowered. Although their jobs are demanding and they often identify strongly with their work, they do not have access to many of the sources of recognition and self-esteem enjoyed by members of professional groups.

Formal Recognition

On-the-job recognition formally sponsored by your facility can have especially powerful effects for caregiving staff. Coming up with ways to recognize your staff can be fun! Use your imagination and creativity. Brainstorm with your team about how they would like to be recognized for their hard work.

Human resources expert Robert L. Desatnick makes some wonderful suggestions in his book *Keep the Customer.* Here are a few of his ideas, drawn from Fortune 500 firms, adapted to the nursing home:

- Run internal contests where staff on different units compete to be the best in some area (e.g., low absenteeism) during a given time period.

- Sponsor "Employee of the Month" and "Unit of the Month" recognition programs.

- Solicit letters of recognition from family members, and display them in the facility's entrance or lounge. Send copies to local media, legislators, and governor's and mayor's offices.

- Publish stories of outstanding service by your staff in your facility newsletter.

- Place a special recognition symbol on an employee's name badge for outstanding job performance.

- Sponsor staff parties and trips.

- Elect a "Rookie of the Month" at a gathering attended by fellow staff, to recognize a new employee for outstanding service.

Informal Recognition

An equally powerful form of recognition is informal recognition—the way that you affirm the contributions that nursing assistants make on a day-to-day basis.

Validate nursing assistants for the good care they give. Make it a habit when interacting with your staff to respond to a job well done by saying, "Thank you." Notice and publicly acknowledge at least one action by a caregiver every day.

Public recognition for good work is just the beginning. When someone does something well, put it in writing. Send a note or letter to a caregiver to show appreciation for outstanding work. This is especially appropriate when a resident or family member reports a positive experience with a caregiver.

Long-term care staff are unsung heroes, but it doesn't have to be that way. Take the time to notice their special contributions in informal and formal ways.

Do's and Don'ts for Informal Recognition

1. **Do mix praise with criticism.** Often, supervisors feel they need to focus on problems. If the staff person who has made a mistake performs the task correctly the other 99% of the time, include that feedback. For example, instead of saying, "This is the second time you're late this week. This is intolerable!" consider saying, "You know, you are usually very responsible about coming on time, and I appreciate that. What's been going on this week?"

2. **Do try to be specific.** Just saying "Great job, keep it up!" will begin to have an insincere ring after a while. Point out exactly what you think was done well. For example: "I noticed that you really took the time to allow Mrs. Watts to dress herself. I know that means a lot to her." Staff will realize that you notice when they do something well.

3. **Don't go overboard.** Always make sure that your positive feedback is genuine. Remember that you need to find a happy medium. If you give too many "pats on the back" for routine tasks, your recognition may lose its effectiveness.

4. **Don't be phony.** Your staff will see right through you if you are not sincere. Ask yourself: Is this really a praiseworthy thing she did, or am I just trying to make her feel good?

CHAPTER 9

Helping Staff Achieve Work/Life Balance

"There is more to life than increasing its speed."
—*Mahatma Gandhi*

Nursing staff often find themselves scrambling to meet their professional and family responsibilities and are torn by these competing demands. This problem can be made worse by the staffing shortage and today's typically busy family life. At some point, everyone has to do a little juggling to manage personal life while maintaining work performance. You may know first-hand how stressful this balancing act can be. As a supervisor, you can provide valuable support to your staff as they perform this daily balancing act.

Recognizing Signs of Personal Problems

People under stress often compound their problems with ineffective or counterproductive strategies, such as smoking, habitual drinking, or overeating. In your leadership role, you can help to educate your staff about stress-reduction strategies that promote health and well-being. (See the tips in Chapter 11 for some ideas.)

Some signs of damaging stress include a sudden change in performance or behavior such as persistent irritability, excessively strong emotions in response to situations, and frequent tardiness or absences.

To offer support, you need to learn more about the underlying problem. However, be sensitive to the fact that some people may not want to discuss personal problems in detail. When talking with a team member about a personal problem, you must be careful not to overstep professional boundaries. Communicate your respect for your staff's privacy, and your desire to help them maintain satisfactory job performance while they deal with other issues.

Addressing Personal Problems

- If your facility has an Employee Assistance Program (EAP), encourage the team member to explore this option. An EAP is a service, often free of charge, that helps employees and their families deal with personal problems, such as eldercare or childcare issues, abusive relationships, drug and alcohol problems, financial difficulties, depression, or personal crises. When suggesting the EAP to a team member, emphasize that you are not making a judgment, accusation, or diagnosis. Your goal is to help the team member better meet his or her job responsibilities.

- A change in schedule or shift might be the answer for someone with temporary problems. Ongoing conflicts between work and family responsibilities may require a switch from full-time to part-time or flex-time. Other team members may agree to help by acccommodating temporary schedule changes.

- A difficult problem may require that your team member take a leave of absence. The Family Medical Leave Act allows full-time employees who have worked for a company for more than one year to take an unpaid leave to deal with serious personal or family health problems or to care for a new child. Some employers also offer unpaid personal leaves for people who have difficulties that do not fall under the provisions of the Family Medical Leave Act. Before discussing this with a team member, consult with the appropriate person in your human resources or personnel department.

As a supervisor, you are a resource to the members of your team, not a sympathetic friend. This doesn't mean that you must be aloof or unfriendly; it means that you become ineffective as a supervisor when you get too involved with a team member's personal problems.

Self-Care Contracts

Professional caregivers have a natural gift for thinking about the needs of others. They are also at risk for stress-related problems arising from their dedication to the care of those they serve. Practicing a structured approach to wellness promotion for you and your staff can reduce this risk.

Faculty at the Norwich University School of Nursing developed a useful tool called the self-care contract, a written statement in which staff members assess their own self-care needs. The self-care contract encourages setting clear and realistic goals to be accomplished within specific timeframes, for example, eight to ten weeks. Items on a self-care contract might include:

- I will exercise 20 minutes a day, at least three times per week.

- I will allow myself at least 30 minutes of solitude per week, time away from work or family responsibilities.

- I will eat and enjoy at least five fruits and vegetables a day.

Writing a self-care contract should be voluntary. However, for those who choose to participate, providing an opportunity for a brief progress check at regularly scheduled staff meetings can be helpful. This promotes the concept of self-care as part of your organizational work culture.

SPOTLIGHT ON . . .

Resources for Life's Stresses

Unfortunately, low-income workers may experience what is known as an "accumulation of disadvantage." The difficulties of making ends meet, finding child care, obtaining reliable transportation, and dealing with family problems are more challenging when a full-time worker has limited financial resources. Some CNAs and other non-professional staff may require concrete help with life problems to become reliable employees who enjoy their jobs.

It's helpful for nurse managers who supervise CNAs to educate themselves about resources available to citizens in their city, county, and state. Local service agencies may be able to provide assistance to employees who are experiencing problems in their personal lives. For example, a CNA may have trouble getting to work because of a car breakdown or change in a bus schedule. A car "loan and repair" program may exist in your county to assist workers with auto repairs or obtaining a used-car loan. Child care councils might help find day care or after-school programs.

An information kiosk placed in a staff lounge or wherever staff can easily access it can be an effective way to disseminate information about local resources. Fill the kiosk with brochures from local agencies and service programs, including transportation, child and elder care, counseling services, and credit assistance. Providing this type of practical information may help reduce absenteeism in your facility by helping your staff to deal with common life challenges.

CHAPTER 10

Dealing with Conflict

"Conflict is the primary engine of creativity and innovation."
—*Ronald Heifetz*

Handling conflict isn't easy. However, conflict is a natural part of human interaction, especially in today's fast-paced, high-pressure health care environments. By setting a positive example, maintaining a professional environment, and recognizing and addressing conflicts before they escalate, you can help your staff to avoid serious pitfalls. The listening and communication skills discussed earlier in this book will help in resolving everyday conflicts and more difficult situations when team members seem hostile and unable to work together. It is important to remember—and to remind your staff—that conflict has a positive side. Respectful disagreements provide an opportunity to learn from others, and to create new and mutually satisfying solutions.

It is natural to react defensively when we feel criticized. Unfortunately, defensiveness sets up barriers to communication, making it more difficult to come up with solutions that meet everyone's needs. Learning to respond to blame and criticism in a less emotional way is an important life skill that can improve both work and personal relationships.

Negotiating Creative Solutions

In your role as a nurse supervisor, you will be called on to resolve conflicts and to negotiate with staff members, residents, and families. Many people find the idea of negotiating frightening, yet it is a skill we use every day without much thought. Negotiations can be conducted over large issues, such as the price of a house, or small issues, such as how to spend a Saturday afternoon. In a nursing facility, as in other work situations, the large issues may involve topics such as assignments, salary, promotions, and time off.

When negotiating large issues, people tend to take rigid positions and become defensive—and to see the other negotiator as an adversary. They also assume that the other person has contradictory needs and wants. Often, one person will leave the negotiation feeling like a "winner" and the other like a "loser." Any bad feelings that result can adversely affect future interactions.

It doesn't have to be this way. Roger Fisher and William Ury of the Harvard Negotiation Project, in the classic book *Getting to Yes,* suggest ways to use negotiation to find creative solutions where all parties win. Their premise is that the two parties should approach the negotiation cooperatively, viewing each other as partners. This is particularly important when the relationship is ongoing.

The authors' advice is to "separate the people from the problems." In other words, it isn't constructive to blame or get angry with the other person. The following steps are helpful in accomplishing this separation:

• Think about and discuss the issue from the other person's perspective.

- Speak about yourself—your needs and the problem's impact on you—rather than about the other person.

- Stay calm in response to emotional outbursts.

- Focus on interests, not positions.

The essence of "getting to yes" is to learn what the other person really wants, look for shared interests, and create options that provide a benefit for both parties.

Putting It Into Practice

The next time you encounter conflict, use the seven steps on the following page to achieve a positive resolution. This process provides a structure that will enable you to listen and understand the issue. Instead of taking an adversarial point of view, affirm the other person's position, agree about the problem and its possible solutions, and discuss a timeframe to solve it. This approach recognizes each of you as partners, and builds on your strengths and resources.

Seven Steps to Resolving Conflict

1. The first step in reaching a solution is to **listen.**

2. Next, let the other person know you **understand** the complaint. That doesn't mean you agree with it, but that you understand it.

3. Give the person an **affirmation.** Mention something related that you honestly admire in the person. It is best if this is something that can help in the specific situation.

4. Once you have identified and agreed on the problem, look for the **needs** behind the problem. Too often people rush to solve the problem before understanding the need behind it.

5. Once you understand what each of you needs, you can work together to find a **solution.** If possible, come up with a list of several solutions that might work.

6. Then, together, **choose one** that meets both of your needs.

7. The last step is to **agree on a specific period of time** to try out the solution and to talk it over again.

CHAPTER 11

Dealing with Your Job Stress

"It's not stress that kills us, it is our reaction to it."
—*Hans Selye*

Stress is unavoidable on the job and in our personal lives. The right amount of stress helps us to stay motivated, meet our responsibilities, and move toward our life's goals. However, overwhelming stress can lead to physical, emotional, and spiritual suffering. As a nurse supervisor, learning to manage your job stress effectively not only contributes to your own success, but it can also help you to guide and support those you supervise.

Surveys have shown that many nurses rate job stress as a top personal health concern. Long hours, staffing shortages, and lack of administrative support are all factors that create stress for professional nurses. Long-term care nurses frequently deal with other potential stresses uniquely related to their work environment. High staff turnover rates, lack of clarity about supervisory roles, and isolation from a network of colleagues all contribute to stress. Nursing home residents are typically older and in declining health. Therefore, nurses who work in this setting must frequently deal with death and dying. Long-term care nurses in supervisory roles may have little management training or experience. The good news is that by learning to manage the inevitable stresses of their jobs, nurses can thrive in the face of all these challenges.

A sure prescription for job stress is a lack of self-confidence. If you feel chronically stressed at work, make an honest self-appraisal of your nursing and supervisory skills, seeking the advice of a trusted mentor, if possible. Do you need to update certain clinical skills? Are you at ease with new computer technology in use at your facility, such as electronic medical records? Would some management training help you to better resolve employee conflicts or communicate more effectively with your staff? Are your time management strategies up to par? Identifying areas of weakness is the first step to eliminating them. Building confidence in your knowledge base and expertise places you on firm footing as a supervisor, helps you to be a better resource to your staff, and reduces a potential source of job stress.

Burnout vs. Compassion Fatigue

Experts are beginning to understand that those who work in the "helping" professions—e.g., nurses, psychologists, emergency responders—are susceptible to a special form of stress known as compassion fatigue. Unlike "burnout," which can happen in any workplace and usually stems from frustration with the organization or "system," compassion fatigue is triggered by the stress of caring. Physiological signs of burnout and compassion fatigue are similar and may include headaches, extreme fatigue, sleep disturbances, and difficulty concentrating. Compassion fatigue and job burnout can coexist.

A hallmark of compassion fatigue is that it affects the quality of care provided to others and to one's self. The phenomenon is characterized by emotional detachment and apparent lack of empathy for others, or at the other extreme, intense over-involvement. Whereas burnout can usually be alleviated by addressing the underlying problem, or by taking a vacation or changing jobs, compassion fatigue persists in spite of these attempts to improve the situation.

Preventing and treating compassion fatigue involves maintaining or reestablishing the boundary between "self" and "other." This is accomplished by understanding the need for specific self-care measures, and following through with them.

- Assess your level of stress periodically. Are you eating and sleeping well? Do you have trouble staying focused on the task at hand? Acknowledging a problem is the first step to its solution.

- Are you in tune with your body? Are you "tied in knots" by the end of the day? Try to incorporate some form of conscious movement in your day, either through gentle stretching exercises, taking a walk, or getting regular massage.

- Incorporate a daily self-care ritual into your routine. This may be as simple as reading a passage from an inspirational book, writing in a journal, or working in your garden.

- Do you have a sense of connection with others? Are you able to ask for help when you need it? Nurses are experts at being there for others but often feel uncomfortable on the receiving end. Learn to recognize and accept your own need for nurturing.

Time-Tested Ways to Reduce Stress

Much of the excess daily stress that we face can be prevented by maintaining a healthy body and a healthy frame of mind. Exercise and striving for a positive, lighthearted outlook on life can go a long way in managing stress. Incorporate these strategies in your daily life, and suggest them to others who are having a difficult time managing stress.

Exercise. If you currently have a regular exercise routine, that's great. If you aren't physically active, start to engage in some sort of regular program of exercise. You don't have to buy an expensive club membership. Try going for brisk walks alone or with a friend, or following along with an aerobics show on television. Be creative and do what you enjoy.

Eat well. It is true that you are what you eat! If you exist on junk food and coffee, stress gains the upper hand. Add healthful foods, such as fruits and vegetables, and cut back on coffee, sugary sodas, and junk food. Vitamins and minerals obtained from a balanced diet give your body what it naturally needs to defend and protect itself.

Get enough sleep. Studies show that many Americans are chronically short of sleep. You probably already know from experience how much sleep you need to perform at your best. Make an effort to regularly get the amount of sleep that is right for you.

Learn to relax. Take "time out" to sit quietly, relax your muscles, and clear your mind. Focused relaxation recharges your system for any difficult or stressful tasks ahead.

Express your feelings. If you feel stressed, talk to a trusted friend who can be your sounding board. Often, problems swirling in your mind seem more manageable when they are spoken out loud.

Lighten up. Try to take life less seriously. Cultivate your inner sense of humor. Do something nice for people in your life. Take the time to enjoy life's little pleasures and surprises.

CHAPTER 12

Humor at Work

"The old man laughed loud and joyously, shook up the details of his anatomy from head to foot, and ended by saying such a laugh was money in a man's pocket, because it cut down the doctor's bills like anything."

—Mark Twain

On first glance at the chapter title, you might wonder what humor has to do with your role as a nurse supervisor. A quick look back in history provides a hint. The word *humor* comes from a Latin word for "moisture," or "liquid." In the Middle Ages, doctors believed that the relative amounts of four humors in the human body determined a person's health and disposition. They reasoned that an imbalance of these substances caused illness or bad temperament. The physician's job was to restore balance to the four humors, thus healing the patient.

The health benefits of humor are being rediscovered, thanks to ongoing research on the effects of humor on the body and mind. The appropriate use of humor has been shown to improve mood, reduce stress and pain perception, and strengthen relationships. Evidence also suggests that experiencing humor may boost the immune system and help to prevent disease.

The Association for Applied and Therapeutic Humor defines therapeutic humor as "any intervention that promotes health and wellness by stimulating a playful discovery, expression or appreciation of the absurdity or incongruity of life's situations." Therapeutic humor differs from comedy in that it is always positive, and never insults, teases, or lacks sensitivity to the feelings of others. Ethnic jokes, sexual innuendo, and put-downs create barriers between people, whereas therapeutic humor brings people together to share in life's joys.

Therapeutic Humor and the Long-Term Care Nurse

Nurses tend to be closely attuned to the needs and feelings of others and can use this gift of sensitivity to bring humor into the workplace to heal the spirit. The observation and assessment skills used every day in the nursing process can be used to assess the receptivity of residents to a bit of lighthearted humor. In your leadership role, you can help to guide your staff in the appropriate use of humor by modeling this behavior for them.

If you are unsure of how to infuse humor into your work as a nurse supervisor, the first rule is to be yourself. Humor can't be forced. Try to be receptive to the little absurdities of life that happen throughout the day, and share them with others. Adding humor to the long-term care facility environment can take many forms. Whether it's a formal "laughter club" organized by the activity department, an informal facility-wide contest for the joke of the day, or the individual efforts of nurses and other staff members spreading joy to others, humor can enrich the lives of residents and staff in surprising ways. Brightening the atmosphere in the long-term care facility where you work can have a "ripple effect," helping to bring cheer and peace to your community and to the world.

When Humor Feels Inappropriate

Many health care workers are familiar with a phenomenon called "gallows humor," a brand of humor that seems to suddenly emerge in the midst of the most tragic circumstances. A patient dies and a frantic search for his dentures ends in a burst of laughter from the nurses' station. In the midst of resuscitation efforts, a nurse gets the giggles at the sight of the chaotic scene. Experts tell us that such reactions are an important "relief valve" that protects us from becoming overwhelmed in emotionally charged situations. In fact, emergency department personnel are particularly experienced with this phenomenon. Obviously, this type of humor is never appropriate in the presence of residents or visiting family members. However, in its place, gallows humor serves a useful purpose and should bring no guilt.

Death and Dying . . . and Humor?

In his book titled *The Courage to Laugh*, Alan Klein asks humorist and former hospice nurse Patty Wooten how she and her fellow staff nurses were able to laugh in the face of so much death in their daily work. Her reply is worth noting: "[Laughter] gives buoyancy so you just don't sink to the bottom. Like a life preserver, it helps keep your head above water so you can still breathe. The heaviness of the situation feels like it can pull you under, like you are drowning, and laughter is like a breath of fresh air that you desperately need."

What long-term care nurse has never felt the heaviness that Patty describes? By the nature of their work, long-term care nurses witness the physical and cognitive decline, and deaths, of residents they have grown to know well, and love. Sharing life's joy through humor can be life-affirming and helps to keep things in perspective. A sense of humor is a healthy tool for dealing with stress and prevents us from becoming emotionally blunted by unpleasant or even tragic circumstances that are common in health care settings.

People who are nearing death are sometimes receptive to humor for the same reasons. Humor shines a light in the darkness, lifts the spirit, and enhances human connections. Engaging in humor with a resident who is terminally ill is not out of the question. In fact, according to Klein, it can often be therapeutic. He suggests starting by asking the person, at a time that seems appropriate, how long it has been since they have laughed, or what sorts of things they have found humorous in the past. The resident may be relieved to know that he or she is not expected to be always sad and tearful, but can enjoy the lighter side of life, too.

Using Humor with Residents

- Know the resident. It takes some time to get a feel for someone's receptivity to humor.

- Keep it positive. Therapeutic humor never gets a laugh at someone else's expense.

- Test the waters with a funny pin on your sweater or a silly prop on the med cart. The resident can choose to pick up on it, or not.

- Create a "humor cart" filled with funny props and silly items. Be creative and involve other staff members in the project.

- Recognize that humor is in the eye of the beholder. Respect the rights of others, who may have different views about what is funny.

- Remember that your primary concern is always the residents' physical and emotional comfort. Fit humor in only where it naturally blends with that goal.

- Make sure residents see your professionalism. In the words of therapeutic nurse humorist Patty Wooten, "You need to let your patients know that you're competent before you let them know you're funny."

CHAPTER 13

Making Diversity Work

"Leadership and learning are indispensible to each other."
—*John R Kennedy*

Today's caregivers come from many backgrounds. Your team may include people of different cultural groups, ages, genders, religions, sexual orientations, life experiences, and races. Generally, diversity adds to the quality of our workplace. However, we must recognize that because people see things from different perspectives, conflicts may arise at times.

Managing diversity means being open to incorporating different styles of problem solving, different attitudes, and different backgrounds into the workplace culture. People on your team must be able to work together, even if their beliefs or backgrounds are not the same. The standard you set will influence the way your team members interact with each other.

Our culture shapes the way we view ourselves, the people around us, the things we value, and the ways we behave. As a nurse manager, learning to appreciate cultural differences does more than prevent hurt feelings; it also improves your ability to supervise and gain the cooperation of your staff.

Culture: What Is It?

Different cultures are made up of various styles of food, clothing, music, art, languages, and rules for dealing with social situations. Whereas culture can be defined by geographic area (for example, Northerners and Southerners), a location can encompass several coexisting cultures (for example, New York City). A good definition of *culture* might be a set of attitudes, beliefs, values, and behaviors shared by a group of people.

As a leader and team builder, you should be aware of the background and culture of your team members. Insensitivity to cultural differences can undermine your efforts to build connections to and within the group. If you witness disrespectful behavior or language, speak separately with the individuals to get a clearer sense of the situation. Bring the issue to your supervisor if the problem seems to be escalating or prevents the team from working together effectively.

Generally speaking, people work to their full capabilities when they feel trusted and safe from intolerance. You can help your staff to reach their potential by showing trust and confidence in their abilities and fostering an atmosphere where everyone is valued.

How Does Diversity Affect Your Staff?

Learning to appreciate cultural differences can help nursing assistants improve their relations with other members of the caregiving team while also helping them to understand behaviors of residents. Nursing home staff report that diversity affects their work in a variety of ways. Here are some of their thoughts on the topic, in their own words:

- Although all of our residents are English-speaking, they come from very different backgrounds. We often have poetry, writing, and reading activities, which most of our residents enjoy. But one resident absolutely does not relate to what we are talking about. Although she is very smart, she grew up on a farm and has a third-grade education. Books were not a big part of her life.
  —*Nursing Assistant from Issaquah, Washington*

- The nursing assistants here are mostly of Hispanic or Anglo-Saxon origin. Any language or cultural barriers have been overcome by personalizing things. Even when new people come in, everyone is very accepting of each other. Once you know the others, you can work better as a team. We're here for one common goal: to take care of the residents.
  —*Nursing Assistant from Rye, New Hampshire*

- We need to take time to explain our different cultures. We have many Italian, Spanish, and Lithuanian residents. When I don't understand one of them I point to my skin and say, "I am a black American" to remind them that we have different backgrounds. I've noticed that Italian-speaking residents are more likely to ask for Spanish-speaking nursing assistants, because the language sounds familiar.
  —*Nursing Assistant from Waterbury, Connecticut*

Chances are, the mix of staff and residents at your facility is comprised of a mix of cultural or ethnic groups. Although these differences can present a supervisory challenge at times, remember that they can also be a

source of strength. Helping your staff to embrace and
appreciate their uniqueness as individuals and as a group
can improve team spirit and lead to better care.

SIX STEPS TO CULTURAL UNDERSTANDING

Below are six steps in the process of understanding cultural
differences:

1. **Denial of Differences.** The attitude "we're all the
   same under the skin" discounts the real differences
   among people from other cultures. This attitude refuses
   to see the differences at all.

2. **Defensiveness.** In this step, differences are
   acknowledged, but one's own point of view is considered
   "right," and other viewpoints are considered "wrong."

3. **Minimizing Differences.** In this step, differences are
   recognized but are granted no importance. This step
   could be called the "So What?" step.

4. **Acceptance.** This step recognizes and appreciates the
   importance of cultural differences.

5. **Adapting to Reality.** Empathy and communication
   skills are used to bridge cultural differences.

6. **Ongoing Learning.** This final step involves a
   sustained respect for others' differences and a growing
   understanding of the skills needed to live and work
   together.

Once you and your staff come to understand the
opportunities that come with diversity, you can use the
differences in cultural and ethnic background to enrich
the relationships among the staff, the residents, and
residents' families.

Fostering Cultural Competency

You may have heard residents say, "We have so many staff from different countries; I don't always understand what they are saying." Sometimes language and accent differences can be complicated for older adults, especially those with hearing impairments. Stereotyping of members of other groups can also be an issue when residents or staff have preconceived notions about—or active prejudices against—other groups.

As a manager, you may find it useful to conduct cultural competence training programs. Some facilities conduct an orientation for new staff; for example, certain Jewish nursing facilities have developed trainings on understanding Jewish life and culture. Nursing homes can develop booklets or flyers about different practices, customs, and rituals. It can be helpful for staff to learn some expressions in other languages. For example, a facility with many Spanish-speaking residents can train staff in common expressions, which can make residents feel more at home.

Studies of cultural competency suggest that staff need good communication and empathy skills to work well in a culturally diverse environment. They need to become comfortable asking about residents' preferences and avoid making assumptions based on that person's cultural background. It is critical for staff to understand and appreciate cultural practices of residents and coworkers that are different from their own. Exploring the similarities of unfamiliar customs can further understanding between individuals and groups of differing cultures.

Tips for Honoring Cultural Differences

- Learn and use some key words of the languages around you.

- Watch how others of the same culture communicate. Observe how members of your own culture relate with one another. Compare the two ways without judging either one better than the other.

- Be sensitive to others' customs, holidays, and religious practices. Express your interest by asking respectful, polite questions. Be prepared to share some of your own customs with them as well.

- Examine the attitudes and beliefs you have about other people. Where did your attitudes and beliefs come from?

- Make a friend from another cultural group.

- When you hear others using stereotypes to describe others, be an advocate for tolerance and understanding.

CHAPTER 14

Performance Management

"The greater danger for most of us lies not in setting our aim too high and falling short; but in setting our aim too low, and achieving our mark."
—*Michelangelo*

Performance management is the process of guiding an organization toward accomplishing its mission. It is both art and science. In long-term care, performance management involves fostering positive working relationships, ensuring compliance with government regulations and facility policies, and finding ways to fairly measure the employees' success in fulfilling their duties.

In many long-term care facilities, senior management establishes performance goals, measures and analyzes the organization's performance as a whole, and sets policies and procedures. But it is the nurse supervisor who is faced with the challenge of managing frontline workers in accomplishing the daily tasks that contribute to the overall mission.

Successful performance management depends on applying basic human resource skills every day, not only at occasional meetings or when problems arise. Although each facility's policies and procedures vary, the basic elements of employee performance management include the following:

1. **Performance planning**—establishing performance goals, objectives, and expectations

2. **Performance monitoring**—observing performance and providing feedback and coaching

3. **Performance appraisal**—formally documenting and delivering feedback to the employee

Performance planning: Having a specific job description for each employee is critical for successful performance planning. Know what performance measurement tools, such as surveys or data collection, are used at your facility and how they are interpreted. Performance goals should be objective, relevant, and measurable, and clearly reflect management goals. For example, if the department is rated on quantity and quality measurements such as timeliness or infection rates, be sure that the performance plans reflect the same criteria.

Performance coaching: As a nurse manager, you need to identify performance gaps and their causes, and implement appropriate action. Focusing on punitive measures to correct poor performance can demoralize your staff, whereas providing thoughtful feedback can motivate employees to improve performance and quality. Remember that feedback is a two-way street. Be open to suggestions and constructive criticism from your staff.

Performance appraisal: When you notice a deficiency, address it right away instead of waiting for the formal performance evaluation session to bring it up. Analyze its cause. Does the employee need more training? Does a policy or procedure need to be clarified or reassessed? Is there a lack of motivation? If performance gaps exist in more than one area, prioritize those that have the greatest impact on resident safety and well-being.

Performance Appraisal

A formal performance appraisal should be conducted after the first six months of employment and no less than annually thereafter, or in accordance with your facility's human resource policies. This is the opportunity for individual performance to be documented and rated, to reward good performance, and to address performance expectations for the upcoming evaluation period. Staff should have an opportunity to provide their own formal response to the appraisal. Many supervisors ask the employee to draft a self-appraisal as a starting point for discussion. The benefit of this approach is that it quickly reveals any differences in viewpoint between staff member and supervisor. Coupled with regular constructive feedback throughout the year, the formal performance appraisal allows for the employee's ongoing growth and development.

The following are some common causes of poor performance and possible remedies:

Problem: Unclear job expectations and lack of performance feedback

Solution: Be sure that employees are aware of job expectations; do not wait for a performance review to clarify job requirements.

Problem: Lack of knowledge or skills

Solution: Provide in-service training or on-the-job mentoring.

Problem: Inadequate facilities, equipment, or supplies

Solution: Failing to invest here is false economy. Have systems in place to address ongoing issues and needs.

Problem: Lack of motivation, recognition, and positive feedback

Solution: Earning a salary is an important motivation to work, but raises and bonuses alone are generally not effective over the long term. Look for other ways to make your staff feel appreciated. One highly successful manager was legendary for feeding her staff at meetings—bagels on Monday morning, pizza at staff meetings, cookies from her kitchen, and a jar of candy on her desk. Providing and sharing food conveys nurturing. It is an effective reward for success, and a comfort in difficult times. If the budget is limited for such expenses, potluck lunches work just as well.

Managing Change: Mergers, management reorganizations, and major policy changes are part of the long-term care landscape, and your staff may have to face one of these major changes at some point in their careers. Although change is inevitable, our response to change determines its effect on us. Those who see change in a positive light—as an opportunity—are more successful than those who approach change with fear and dread.

With this in mind, nurse supervisors can set the tone for employees by modeling a positive attitude toward an impending change. Share stories of unexpected change that resulted in advancement, reward, or positive results. Accept the fact that some people fear change. Speak privately to anyone who appears unduly stressed, and suggest stress management counseling, if appropriate.

A Personal Touch

Frontline staff members often feel that their efforts are overlooked. Simply greeting employees with a smile—and using their names—demonstrates that you are interested in them and that you are approachable. As a nurse supervisor, find ways to recognize the contributions of individual staff members to the organization's goals. Employee-of-the-month award programs, periodic newsletters, memos, and e-mails that announce staff achievements all provide important positive reinforcement. Try to remain visible and accessible to your staff. Informal praise—saying "good job" or "well done," when appropriate—can go a long way to helping employees feel appreciated. Model a positive attitude and demonstrate the same problem-solving and communication skills that you would like to see in your staff.

Staff Meetings

Staff meetings should be well-planned to make best use of employee time. Always prepare a written agenda. Remember that having too few meetings—or too many—can be counterproductive. Staff meetings help to build a cohesive team that pulls in the same direction. These face-to-face sessions allow everyone to hear the same message and to better understand the current issues affecting the residents, staff, and the facility. Weekly lunch meetings can be a helpful and informal way to stay in tune with staff and their concerns.

It is a safe bet that everyone on your staff prefers a happy workplace, so make this a conscious goal. Devote a portion of regular staff meetings for airing concerns or making suggestions for improving the workplace atmosphere. Empower staff to develop their own solutions and to report back to the group. This approach helps team members develop problem solving and conflict management skills, as they practice resolving issues on their own.

CHAPTER 15

Everyday Ethics in Long-Term Care

"We do not act rightly because we have virtue or excellence, but we rather have those because we have acted rightly."
—*Aristotle*

Ethics can be thought of as a group of principles containing an element of morality—right versus wrong—that guide behavior. Ethics governs virtually all kinds of human interaction, from international relations to seemingly minor daily decisions, such as whether or not to tell a convenience store clerk that she gave you too much change.

Ethics influences every area of health care delivery and clinical practice. Health care administrators must decide how to allocate funds for staffing, equipment, and supplies, balancing concern for the financial health of the organization with the needs of those they serve. Physicians must consider risk versus benefit when deciding treatment options. Nursing supervisors make everyday ethical decisions when they decide how to juggle their numerous responsibilities, or whether or not to permit a nursing home resident to smoke.

Ethics in the health care environment—also known as bioethics—often involves profound life and death issues such as artificial nutrition and hydration, "do not resuscitate" orders, and end-of-life pain management. However, the "ethics of the ordinary" deserves as much attention, particularly in long-term care settings, as this realm of ethics influences the quality of life for nursing home residents every day.

"Everyday ethics" is embedded in the central ethical principles set forth in the American Nurses Association "Code of Ethics for Nurses," namely, the patient's right to self-determination, respect for human dignity and choices, and preservation of confidentiality and privacy. Everyday ethics involves the seemingly ordinary decisions caregivers make throughout their workday, often while balancing the conflicting priorities and interests of different people.

Some facets of nursing home life are beyond the control of the nursing supervisor and staff. However, a heightened awareness of the scope and importance of "everyday ethics" will enhance your ability to ensure that residents' dignity and quality of life are preserved. Although many nursing home rules and routines serve a useful purpose, they sometimes conflict with the desires of individual residents. Flexibility and creativity are keys to resolving these conflicts, with the goal of offering a meaningful choice to residents whenever possible.

Everyday Ethics in Practice

For most residents, entering a nursing home means making a variety of lifestyle adjustments. Giving up a houseful of cherished belongings, adjusting to the loss of a spouse, or grappling with declining health and mobility are all common scenarios facing older adults who are entering a nursing home. Everyday ethics involves helping residents to achieve the highest possible quality of life by offering as much choice as possible about the things that matter to them. It means allowing residents as much control over their environment as is feasible.

Showing respect for the resident's personal space is one way to do this. Knocking before entering a resident's room is a basic courtesy, but how many staff members wait for a response before dashing inside? Similarly, asking permission before rearranging the resident's belongings on a bedside table demonstrates respect and consideration by placing the resident's dignity and right to control his or her environment ahead of staff convenience.

Preserving a resident's dignity means that every request must be considered and honored if at all possible. If a resident's wishes cannot be accommodated, for example, when they conflict with the rights of others, providing a reasonable explanation of why they cannot be accommodated sends the message that the resident is a worthy person.

Decision-Making Capacity

A resident's capacity to make decisions for himself or herself is a central issue in everyday ethics, as in all health care decisions. The ability to make an informed choice requires some level of understanding of the decision's consequences, and this capacity may fluctuate with medical status, cognitive ability, stress level, and even the time of day. Most people, including cognitively impaired residents, have some degree of decision-making capacity.

Capacity is not "absolute," that is, it can be thought of as a sliding scale—when the risk associated with a decision is high, a higher degree of capacity (that is, understanding) is required to make the decision. For example, a cognitively impaired resident may be unable to comprehend the implications of consenting to a new treatment, but still be able to choose what to have for dessert.

Suppose that a resident wants to smoke cigarettes. Does he understand the health implications of his decision? Does the resident understand the facility's fire and safety policies with regard to smoking? Is he able to access designated smoking areas? If he needs supervision, are there enough staff available to provide it? Where does the facility's obligation to preserve the resident's well-being enter into the picture? What effect will the resident's decision to smoke have on other residents and staff? Often, the answers to what is essentially an ethical situation are not easy or simple.

For virtually all ethical dilemmas, an "ethics case study" approach, with input of other members of the health care team, the resident's family, and the resident, is the best way to proceed: What is the issue? Is it a legal or ethical one? Who are the stakeholders? Do we need additional information? What are the options and the risks, benefits, burdens, and consequences of each option? Can we compromise? Once a decision is made, it is essential to revisit the issue later to evaluate the decision and its outcome.

The Code of Ethics offers the following:

- limitation of individual rights must always be considered a serious deviation from the standard of care, justified only when there are no less restrictive means available to preserve the rights of others and the demands of justice.

Assessing Decision-Making Capacity

Determining a resident's capacity to make decisions requires careful observation and documentation about the kinds of decisions the resident does make, whether or not they seem appropriate, given the context, and the resident's ability to follow simple-to-complex directions.

No single test can determine decision-making capacity. The Mini Mental Status Exam—a short series of questions and tasks that assesses orientation, recall, attention, reasoning, and language—is a helpful screen for cognitive impairment but cannot determine decision-making capacity.

One good approach is similar to the method used for obtaining informed consent:

- First, determine if the resident is able to make any kind of decision at all.

- Explain the present decision that needs to be made.

- Ask the resident to repeat it back to you in his or her own words. Encourage questions.

- Assess for the resident's appreciation of the facts and context of the situation.

- Ask the resident his or her decision and, in his or her own words, why the resident made that choice.

- Repeat the process a few hours later, and look for consistency in response and logic.

While nursing home residents have varying cognitive abilities and capacity for decision making, nearly all are still able to make choices about some aspects of their lives. By recognizing how to apply the ethical principles of self-determination and respect for human dignity in their everyday interactions with residents, and by modeling this behavior for other staff members, the nurse supervisor contributes immeasurably to the residents' quality of life.

DECISION MAKING CAPACITY

Decision making capacity is a *clinical determination* and refers to a person's present ability to make reasonable decisions regarding health care concerns.

COMPETENCE

Competence is a *legal term* that refers to a person's ability to make reasonable life decisions. Competence is determined through legal court proceedings.

Ethics and Dementia

Cognitively impaired residents may be unable to completely express their wishes. While offering too many choices can create confusion for a resident with dementia, it is still possible to show respect For example, asking which direction he would like to take during a stroll down the hall, or providing a choice of two snacks conveys concern for the resident's preferences. When dementia is advanced, preserving familiar sights, sounds, and scents in the resident's room is a sensitive yet simple demonstration of respect for the resident.

Everyday ethics also means discovering each resident's uniqueness—his past accomplishments and interests, what is important to him today, and his wishes for the future. Getting to know residents is one of the greatest rewards of working in a geriatric setting, and making this effort honors these men and women. Encouraging your staff members to deepen their knowledge about individual residents increases the likelihood that caregivers will be able to offer meaningful choices based on the resident's personal values.

Bibliography

Covey, Steven. (2005). *The 8th Habit: From Effectiveness to Greatness.* New York: Free Press.

Desatnik, Robert L. (1993). *Managing to Keep the Customer.* San Francisco, CA: Jossey-Bass.

Farber-Post, Linda, Blustein, Jeffrey, and Neveloff Dubler, Nancy. (2007). *Handbook for Health Care Ethics Committees.* Baltimore, MD: The Johns Hopkins University Press.

Fisher, Roger, and Ury, William. (1991). *Getting to Yes: Negotiating Agreement Without Giving In.* New York: Penguin.

Klein, Allen. (1998). *The Courage to Laugh.* New York: Tarcher/Putnam.

Meador, Rhoda, Schumacher, Martin, and Pillemer, Karl. (2001). *The Expert CNA's Illustrated Guide to Documentation.* Clifton Park, NY: Delmar/Cengage Learning.

Parker, G.M. (2008) Team Players and Teamwork: New Strategies for the Competitive Enterprise, Second Edition. San Francisco, CA: John Wiley and Sons.

Pillemer, Karl. (1996). *Solving the Frontline Crisis in Long-Term Care: A Practical Guide to Finding and Keeping Quality Nursing Assistants.* Somerville, MA: Frontline Publishing.

Sullivan-Marx, Eileen M., and Gray-Micelli, Deanna, Editors. (2008). *Leadership and Management Skills for Long-Term Care.* New York: Springer Publishing.